Get Thin For Life!
Easiest, Safest, Most Effective ways to KEEP the Weight off for GOOD!

By
Jason Teichner, CHHP, CN, CHT

TABLE OF CONTENTS

Introduction

INTRODUCTION

For the past several decades, and especially the last few decades, trying to maintain an ideal weight has been a huge challenge for hundred of millions of people worldwide. The US seems especially prone to gaining weight and not being able to take it or keep it off. Believe it or not, there are actually only a FEW reasons for this, not several, all of which I will go over in this book. My goal in writing this book is two-fold. Number one, to make it so that you figure out exactly why YOU have been struggling to get and stay at your ideal weight, including going over various health conditions. Number two, to give you all of the tools you will ever need to get to and stay at your ideal weight FOR LIFE!

I will ALWAYS tell the truth as I see it as to why people are overweight (and unhealthy in general). I've written this book under the assumption that you want help with your weight challenges, and sometimes that means being brutally honest about what's really going on with your body and mind, why you do the things that you do, and how to fix it. If you happen to be one of the millions of people who haven't been able to lose weight and keep it off due to a health condition, we will go over all of that as well and how to fix it. To your health and happiness; Let's walk this path together!

Jason Teichner, CHHP, CN, CHT

CHAPTER ONE
The History of Dieting

Fad diets seem to have been around since around 1558, with Lord Byron's "The Art of Living Long". In the book, Byron describes what he felt was the key to losing weight, potatoes flattened and drenched in vinegar. The vinegar was supposed to break up the carbs in the potatoes and speed up metabolism.

In the 19th century, we had our first introduction to low-carb diets, with Dr. Jean-Anthelme Brillat-Savarin, a French physician, followed by William Banting's book in 1863.

In the late 1800's, Horace Fletcher, an American businessman, came up with the 'chewing craze', where he insisted that no matter what a person ate, as long as he/she chewed the food at least 100 times, no weight could be gained, as the food would be turned into liquid.

In 1918, Dr. Lulu Hunt Peters wrote "Diet and Health- With Key to the Calories", a Best Seller, in which she urged women not to eat more than 1200 calories in a day, and as a result they would lose weight. This is when the concept of calorie counting began.

In the 1930's, Dr. William Hay introduced the concept of food combining. There are certain foods when combined together, Hay said, that would make you gain weight, whereas other foods when combined would allow you to lose weight.

The cabbage soup diet came onboard in the 1950's, although who specifically came up with it appears to be unknown.

Dr. Robert Atkins came up with a diet in the 1960's where only fat, protein, and vegetables were allowed. Any simple carb (starch or sugar) would make you gain weight while all other foods would make you lose weight. In 1972, he published his first book, "Dr. Atkins' Diet Revolution". This was followed up by his "New Diet Revolution" in 2002. Since Atkins' dieting suggestions, I don't even need to tell you how many fad diets have popped up since then. Most of you have heard of many of them and possibly even tried a good number of them.

Of all the above diets mentioned, and the ones not mentioned, there is definitely some type of issue I have with each and every one of them. Some are nutrient deficient, some are very rough on your liver and kidneys, some make you starve, only to binge later. In other words, they're all either not safe, don't work, or work for awhile and then stop working. I'm sure most of you would agree with me in your own experience with dieting, otherwise you wouldn't have picked up this book, right?

Why don't they work? Even more permanent so-called lifestyle changes many of you may have adopted are STILL not allowing you to lose weight. WHY IS THAT!? Those are the things we will go over in the next chapter.

CHAPTER TWO

Why am I not Losing Weight!? Mental & Physical Conditions
Let's begin with another assumption.. yeah, yeah, I know what 'they say' about assumptions. I'm going to assume that whether or not you actually do have a health condition, mental or physical, that is keeping you from getting to your ideal weight, once you've read though this book you will no longer use it as an excuse. This is because I will be going over most of the common conditions, many of which can be combined (I'll explain later), as to why you may not be losing weight. Of course if you don't actually have a health condition, then the 'no excuses' rule goes without saying.
The first thing we all need to know is that the mind and body work as one. Each is fully connected to the other. Next, it is a combination of the nervous system (starting in the brain), the endocrine system (the glands, and hormones that are produced from those glands), and the digestive system, that can cause people to not be able to lose weight. All three systems mentioned above are connected. Now, if you're just simply one of those people who knows you eat too much and just can't stop, we'll address that issue as well.

The Nervous System
The nervous system begins in the brain and travels throughout the entire body. It is responsible for all communication throughout the body. Our thoughts turn into feelings, and our feelings turn into actions; in this case the action is telling our neurons (nerve cells, which are the major part of our nervous system) how to communicate with the body at that given time. What's the connection between our nervous and digestive systems? For starters, around 95% percent of the neurotransmitter serotonin is produced in our digestive tract! Ever heard the term, 'nervous stomach'? That's why! The good news is that by changing our thoughts, we can change our feelings, thereby changing our communication pattern throughout the body. This takes practice. At first, we may, at least for a while, need to accept our thoughts but change the feelings that our thoughts turn into, thereby changing the communication.

The autonomic nervous system is the division that includes the neurons. It is divided into two parts: the sympathetic and the parasympathetic. The sympathetic is responsible for our 'fight or flight' response. The body does not know the difference between real danger and perceived danger, so when we are under chronic stress, our sympathetic division becomes overactive, causing our adrenal glands (part of our endocrine system) to pump out too much adrenaline (which speeds up our metabolism temporarily), and then have to make up for it by producing too much cortisol (which slows down our metabolism). Both hormones in excess are not good for us, as number one, it wears out our adrenal glands, making us chronically tired. Number two, when we're in fight or flight mode, our blood is rushing to protect our vital organs for survival instead of going to our digestive system to break down the food we've eaten. This causes food to store in our intestinal tract, causing weight gain. So here we have both cortisol and unbroken down food both creating weight gain. The longer we live like this, the more weight we gain (not to mention the chronic fatigue as well).

The Endocrine System
The endocrine system comprises of all of our glands and the hormones those glands produce. As we said before, the nervous, endocrine, and digestive systems all all connected. Usually our nervous system goes out of whack, causing our endocrine system to go out of whack, which causes our digestive problems. There are cases where the order can be flipped, but in all cases they are all connected, and if you let one be off for long enough, it will eventually cause the other systems to become problematic as well. Most of us have already heard how an underactive thyroid can cause a slowing of our metabolism, which will cause us to hold onto weight. This is way more basic than all of what's really going on in our bodies. Remember, a thyroid issue, just like any other one issue you can think of, as always just a symptom of a larger issue. We'll get a little more into specific names later in the chapter. What I can

say is no matter what you have going on, there IS a natural way to address it, and that's exactly what I'm here to help you do.

First, I will tell you to ask your doctor to do a full thyroid and adrenal panel, not just what is shown in the generic CBC and Chemistry panel. Many doctors will simply look at TSH (Thyroid Stimulating Hormone), which the pituitary gland sends to the thyroid, and T4, one of the basic thyroid hormones, and determine that if they are both in range, then there is no need to do any further testing. There are many cases where you can have some type of thyroid issue that does not show up in the basic bloodwork. A full thyroid panel will also show antibodies, which when abnormal may indicate one of a few types of autoimmune thyroid conditions. The same is true with the adrenal glands. The bloodwork will usually just show the blood cortisol level, when there could be abnormalities in the saliva and/or urine. Also, a full adrenal panel will also show adrenaline, ACTH (comes from the pituitary to the adrenals), and other hormones. I would suggest that if your regular doctor won't do further testing, request to be referred to an Endocrinologist (gland and hormone doctor).

Even though I'll be mentioning certain specific endocrine conditions, I would highly suggest if you'd like to read even more about them, that you get one of the many thyroid and adrenal conditions books that are out there which discuss those conditions more in detail and how to address them naturally. I will have a list of a few of them that I recommend at the end of the book. There are others besides those as well.

What I CAN promise is that I WILL address what you can do to lose weight if you do have or suspect you have a thyroid or adrenal condition in the following chapters. In addition, in rare cases there can also be a pituitary issue and/or a hypothalamus issue. I would at least bring that up to your doctor, so they will do further testing if they feel the need. As I said, those are a lot more rare, but I feel I'd be shortchanging you if I didn't at least mention those possibilities.

Finally, if you would like to see me as a personal client, I can go into further detail with you and your specific conditions. My contact info is at the end of this book. As I mentioned earlier, there are a few common endocrine conditions I'll be going over.

The Digestive System

The digestive system is comprised of the salivary glands, pharynx, esophagus, stomach, gallbladder, liver, pancreas, small intestine, and large intestine (or colon), which consists of the cecum, appendix, rectum, and anus. Also, it is crucial to note that the digestive and immune system go hand in hand, as 70-80% of our immune system is in our digestive system. Now you know why it's so important it is to keep your digestive system clean and healthy.

Your mouth down to your pancreas all produce enzymes to help break down your food, and your intestines produce good bacteria to keep bad bacteria, viruses, fungus, mold, parasites, and other invaders from building up in your system. All of these portions need a specific PH, not too acidic and not too alkaline, to thrive and do their jobs properly. It's when these portions, especially the organs, become too acidic (common) or too alkaline (uncommon) that they will allow these 'invaders' to pop up in your digestive system, making it much harder for it to function properly. It is at this time that we begin holding onto food and not being able to eliminate it properly, creating weight gain, among other problems, like getting sick more often, including potential autoimmune digestive issues, such as Crohn's. This eventually will also affect the endocrine system, sometimes creating autoimmune issues there, such as Hashimoto's (thyroid), and then the brain. This is why I stated earlier that all three of these systems are connected. It can also contribute to lupus (a whole body autoimmune illness).

What we eat directly determines whether our body is acidic, alkaline, or neutral. Most of us eat way too many of the wrong foods that create too much acidity in the body, thus contributing to illness and weight gain. We will get into foods in the next two chapters. In order to test your PH levels, I highly suggest you go to a health food store and get some PH strips. Test your saliva and urine. Saliva should be tested first thing in the morning before eating or drinking anything. Spit into the sink a few times to get rid of any 'old' saliva from the night before, then spit onto the PH strip. Your saliva ideally should be somewhere between 6.5 and 6.8. If you're lower than 6.5, you're too acidic; and if you're above 6.8 (rare because of how most of us eat), then you're too alkaline. Next, test your urine. Again, this is first thing in the morning.

Try to let as much of the urine out as possible before going on the strip; in other words, towards the end of the stream. Ideally your urine PH should be between 6.3 and 6.6. Again here, it is way more common for a person's urine to be too acidic, although I've seen a number of people with urine that is too alkaline. This is usually due to eating foods that create too much ammonia in the body which gets excreted in the urine. By altering your diet as suggested in the following chapters, this along with any other PH imbalance can be corrected.

Low Body Temperature

Low body temperature is the most underrated and least talked about contributor to disease, including weight gain. Low body temperature creates major issues in our digestive system, as well as throughout the body. This is because when our body temperature is below 98.2, it can not produce enough digestive enzymes to breakdown our food properly, and it can not produce enough systemic enzymes to break down tissue. When the tissue builds up, it creates pain in the body, and of course when there aren't enough digestive enzymes, it causes food buildup, which creates invaders in our system and weight gain. Let me be very clear. In my opinion, low body temperature is the NUMBER ONE contributor to disease! It is low body temperature that creates endocrine and brain issues from poor digestion and poor tissue breakdown.

So, here comes the obvious million dollar question: what causes low body temperature? Well, two things: (1) Chemicals (including heavy metals) in our food, water, and environment. (2) STRESS!!! Now, if you were going to ask the question of why all of these issues, including low body temperature, have popped up and gotten worse over the last 20 years, there's your answer! First, more and more chemicals are being put into our food, water, and environment. Second, we are more stressed than ever before. So, that means we need to cleanse our bodies, eat healthier, more organic foods, and destress!

Eventually, low body temperature reeks havoc on our whole body, including our thyroid, adrenal, pituitary, and hypothalamus glands, which keeps our temperature too low, as those are the glands that help regulate body temperature. They can't do their job of that when we keep eating more chemicals and heavy metals, and when we continue to be under stress (fight/flight mode). Then it simply becomes a vicious cycle. So, how do you know if you have low body temperature? First thing in the morning, before eating or drinking anything, take your temperature orally. Ideally, it should be between 98.2 and 98.6. If it's below 98.2, that means your body is not producing enough digestive and systemic enzymes. Of course if it's too high, we know that means your body is fighting something off. In that case, you would re-take it in a week or so.

So, I'm sure once again you're now asking, how the heck to I fix this!? And to that I say, 'hang on, it's all coming up in the following chapters.'

Further Testing
It is crucial, in my opinion, to seek out a Naturopathic Doctor (since regular doctors won't do it, or their tests for these are not reliable),

and get tested, at the very least, for gluten sensitivity (which is Celiac in severe cases), a full food sensitivity panel, heavy metals, mold, candida, parasites, and leaky gut syndrome. This way you will have a baseline on what needs to be cleansed and restored in your body. These conditions are now common, unfortunately, due to the way food is now processed, what's in our food, our water, and our environment.

CHAPTER THREE

What, When, and How to Eat (and not eat)

Prior to getting fully into this chapter, I need to mention a couple of things. First, in part of the chapter, I will be going over foods that are good for weight loss, as well as ones that are bad weight loss. Although highly accurate, this is a general guideline. Every person metabolizes different foods differently. I highly suggest if you want to know the exact foods you should be eating based upon your specific metabolic type, go to: www.metabolictypingonline.com and pay the 50 bucks to get your exact metabolic blueprint. You will be asked a series of questions, and based on your answers, you will get a download of exactly what you should and should not be eating. This list is true for you not only for weight loss, but also for overall health and so you will feel energetic, as opposed to tired, and have a healthy digestive system, as opposed to having any further digestive issues.

Now, some of you may be asking, what about my blood type? Isn't that important too? The answer is yes; however, your metabolic type is much more detailed and tailor made for you specifically than just your blood type. Having said that, I still do suggest (if you haven't already) that you read "Eat Right 4 Your Type" by Dr. Adamo, which talks about what to eat and not eat based on your blood type. This way, you can cross reference what he says, what your metabolic type test says, and what I say, to find the very best program for you.

Finally, I also suggest looking up Dr. Joel Fuhrman at www.drfuhrman.com He developed a very good food pyramid of his own, as well as the ANDI score, which measures the micronutrient density of foods in relation to their calories. The higher amount of micronutrients in the food with a lower amount of calories, the higher the ANDI score, and the healthier it is, according to Dr. Fuhrman. I highly suggest using his food pyramid as a guideline for healthy eating, as opposed to any of the others out there. I had the pleasure of hearing Dr. Fuhrman speak live and in person.

Before I get into what foods are 'good', 'bad' or 'neutral', keep in mind this is a weight loss book, so although most of these foods are as such across the board, I am primarily focusing on whether these foods are 'good', 'bad', or 'neutral' in regards to weight loss specifically.

'What' to eat (and not eat)
Fats & Oils-
Good: Coconut, palm, almond, avocado, olive, safflower, sunflower, flax (don't eat if you have thyroid issues), hemp, chia, fish
Bad: Canola, lard, beef, pork, butter, margarine, rapeseed, milk, any hydrogenated or partially hydrogenated oils (these are trans-fats)
Neutral: Walnut, peanut, macadamia, hazelnut, brazil nut, pecan, soybean
Note: This is not as simple as Monounsaturated, polyunsaturated, and saturated. There are both good and bad fats in each of those three categories.
Proteins-
Good: Black beans (beans can be classified as a protein or carb), pinto beans, black eyed peas, navy beans, walnuts (nuts and seeds can be classified as a protein, carb, or fat), almonds, pecans, sunflower seeds, eggs (not more than 7 per week), fish, plain yogurt with active probiotics (good bacteria)

Bad: Beef, pork, whole milk, cheese (except occasional string cheese is fine), starchy or large beans

Neutral: kidney beans, white beans, peanuts, all other beans not listed above, chicken, turkey, brazil nuts, hazel nuts, all other nuts not listed above

Carbs-

Good: Grapefruit, apples, leafy greens, broccoli and all other cruciferous   vegetables (don't eat if you have an underactive thyroid), lemons, limes, pineapple, plums, brown rice, quinoa, oats, wheat (unless you have gluten sensitivity or Celiac), stevia, xylitol (technically not carbs; these are healthy sweeteners since they are natural: stevia comes from a plant, and xylitol is found in various fruits, grains, and the birch tree- and contain no carbs)

Bad: Grapes, dried fruits, bananas, honeydew melon, guava, passion fruit, mango, carrots (except purple), butternut squash, white rice, potatoes, bread, pasta, anything with flour, white sugar, cooked honey, cooked agave nectar, any kind of corn syrup, especially high fructose corn syrup, any artificial sweetener (technically not a carb, but will eventually give you a carb 'backlash' and negatively affect your pancreas' ability to produce insulin, as well as affect your liver and kidneys, since your body doesn't know what to do with it)

Neutral: Other squash not listed above, other melons not listed above, amaranth, buckwheat, other grains not listed above, raw sugar, raw honey, raw agave nectar, palm sugar, coconut sugar

Note: This is of course not a full list, just a guideline. This is because, as I said, the best way for you to know which foods are good and bad for you specifically is to go to www.metabolictypingonline.com and answer the questions it asks about YOU. Of course you can also contact me if you have further questions about any specific food. My contact info is at the end of this book. Finally, all natural foods eaten should always be Certified Organic, especially the ones with no skin or a thin skin. The pesticides sprayed on foods are a slow killer for us when we eat them often. As mentioned above, they contribute to many diseases.

Now, a word on GMO's (Genetically Modified Organisms). GMO's occur when spores of a certain crop contaminate another crop, creating a hybrid that our body does not recognize as real food. Then hybrids keep creating other hybrids, and each time this is done, the food becomes less and less of an actual food, due to the change in its molecular structure. This now creates, among other things, a lack of enzymes, so the food does not break down properly in our bodies. There are also several claims of this being done on purpose, due to the fact that if it wasn't done, there wouldn't be enough food to feed our population. If a food is Certified Organic, it is automatically non-gmo. At the very least, if there are times where eating organic is not possible, make certain you are getting foods that are non-gmo. GMO's in foods contribute to more diseases than we can count. Our body simply does not know how to process them when they get in our system, and will therefore hang on to them. They will then continue to store in our body, and they do not have the component of 'real food' according to our body, so they won't break down properly, eventually reeking havoc on on our cells and organs, even changing the molecular structure of our cells.

'When' to Eat

One again here, the following advice of when to eat pertains ONLY to weight loss. There are other reasons, as it pertains to overall health, where you would not want to eat like this. The following way to eat can actually make your body more acidic, thereby creating more issues in your body overall; make acid reflux (and other health conditions connected to acid reflux) worse (as you'll be telling your stomach to produce acid more often than normal). This way of eating (below) will help you lose weight, but it should only be done until you're at your ideal weight. At that point, the 5   small meals per day about every 3 hours suggestion (below) should be brought down to 4 medium meals about every four hours. That, plus following the other suggestions in my book, you will be able to maintain your ideal weight while eating less often during the day. As far as the food types you'll want to combine, that will be in the 'how to eat' section. So, with that, here it goes: In order to lose weight the quickest, you'll want to eat small meals 5 times per day, or once about every 3 hours. Ideally, you'll want to exercise (details in next chapter) upon awakening, then eat your first small meal right afterward. If you choose not to exercise in the morning, your first meal should be upon awakening. What you do upon awakening will set your metabolic rate for that day. This will speed up your metabolism so you will lose more weight faster, including burning more carbs, fats, and proteins faster. Eating small meals 5 times per day, or once about every 3 hours, will train your body into thinking you will keep eating constantly, so it will therefore keep your metabolism at the highest rate possible. Also, do not eat within 2 hours of going to bed at night. Finally, drink no more than 4 oz of water with each meal, as drinking too much water will neutralize your stomach acid and your food will not break down properly. The majority of your water should be drunk between meals and should ideally be around ½ oz per pound of body weight in total through the day. So a 200 LB person should aim for around 100 oz of water per day, in total; but not more, as it can put too much pressure on the kidneys and throw your electrolytes out of balance. Of course you'll be adjusting the amount of water you drink as you're losing weight.

'How' to Eat

First, one of the more important things on how to eat, is to eat slowly, chewing your food into as much of a liquid as possible, while relaxed. This accomplishes two things: First, your food will be broken down so your digestive organs do as little work as possible, because your food is already pretty well broken down. Secondly, when your body is relaxed, it will focus the blood going to to digestive organs, as opposed to other areas, as your body will know that it's time to eat. Also, by the blood going to your   digestive organs, it allows those organs to work at full capacity in digesting your food.

Now, as far as food combining, keep in mind this is once again a general rule of thumb and that everyone is different in how they process food. I strongly urge if you want more specific information on food combining, that you read one of the food combining books I suggest at the end of this book.

Having said that, here it goes: Each one of your small meals should have some good fat, some good protein, and some good carbs in it. The other two categories of food help assimilate and metabolize the other category of food. For example, one of your meals can have ½ cup of plain yogurt (protein), with a half of an avocado (fat), and a half of an apple (carb). This should also give you a good idea of around how small each of your 5 meals should be. As far as the rest of your meals, you can go off of my list (earlier, under 'good' fats, carbs, and proteins), and combine them anyway you want. Again, please go to www.metabolictypingonline.com and do the metabolic test on the site to see further of which foods are good for you. It will even give you a chart of which foods you should combine. Again, if you want even more info after that, then you can read one of the suggested food combining books. I do find a lot of people who can simply look at my list and figure out all the foods they should be combining, as they get the general idea from just that. Others may need some additional guidance, and that's ok. As always, if you have any further specific questions on which foods you should be combining, feel free to contact me using my contact info at the end of this book.

CHAPTER FOUR
Nutritional Supplements That Actually Work
In this chapter, just like the last one, the best, safest supplements for weight loss will be focused on the most. However, I will also, as

promised, go over excellent supplements for helping to restore the endocrine system (thyroid, adrenals, pituitary, hypothalamus, etc), as well as supplements to help restore the acid/alkaline (PH level) balance in the body, some supplements for restoring the digestive system, and some for helping brain function. Now, for those of you who are saying, 'Jason, based on what you said about the brain, endocrine, and digestive systems all being connected, isn't there something out there that can, over time, help to restore that whole brain/endocrine/digestive connection in just one supplement?' Ah, excellent question my little grasshoppers. I can say, with great excitement, why yes there is! I actually just discovered it recently, and we will get to that in a bit. Finally, I will throw in a few supplements that I believe just about everyone should be taking. Of course, if you have further questions on any other supplements and how they may help you with your specific health condition, you can contact me, using the info at the end of this book, and we can chat a bit and set up a personal session.

•Now would be as good a time as any for my disclaimer: Be sure and speak to your medical doctor or other licensed health practitioner and get their blessing before trying any of my suggestions. The statements and suggestions I mention in this book, including but not limited to the foods and supplements, have not been evaluated by the Food and Drug Administration and are not intended to diagnose, treat, cure, or prevent any disease.

First, different supplements help in different ways to help people lose weight. Some help break down fat, some help break down carbs, some help break down protein, some help speed up metabolism, and some do two or more of those things. I will be mentioning what each one of them does as I go over it. One type of supplement you will not hear me talking about is caffeine or anything with caffeine in it (except the little in green tea), such as guarana, yerba mate, ephedra (illegal in most states), and others. This is because: they wear out your adrenal glands after a while making you 'crash' when you come off of them; they only work for a month or so, until your body gets used to them, and then they stop working, and if you want them to continue to work you'll have to keep uping your dose; caffeine is not safe in high amounts over a long period of time as it strips your body of trace minerals creating mineral deficiencies, such as iron, magnesium, calcium, potassium, copper, zinc, and others. Remember, caffeine is a drug and I do not recommend drugs for health. Overall, just as a general rule, I don't recommend more than 200mg of caffeine per day (about two 6 oz cups of fairly strong coffee; or a little over two espresso shots). Also, any coffee you drink should always be organic, as coffee plants and cherries (raw beans) are among the most pesticide sprayed crops that exists.

Weight Loss Supplements

Garcinia Cambogia: There's been a lot of craze about this supplement lately. Garcinia comes from a type of bitter orange fruit which grows in southern Africa, parts of Asia, Australia, and Polynesia. Garcinia can help with speeding up metabolism, blocking some fat from fully absorbing, and suppressing appetite. The negatives of garcinia is that it can create acid reflux, or make it worse, as it is acidic to the stomach. Also, it can mimic the jittery feeling of having too much caffeine, even though there's no actual caffeine in it. This supplement works, but use it with caution and start with a smaller dose in case it causes those side effects in you. Further, garcinia should not be taken for more than about three months at a time under any circumstances, as it will eventually make the body too acidic. If you really feel you need another cycle, give your body about a six week break before the next 3 month cycle. The normal dose is 500mg twice a day with 50% (250mg) of Hydroxycitric Acid (HCA), as it is the HCA that helps with weight loss. Do not exceed that dose.

Green Tea Extract: Green tea extract is a great weight loss supplement, as it helps speed up metabolism and helps burn loose fat (the fat that is already a gel, ready and waiting to be released). The main ingredient that helps with fat burning and metabolism in green tea is Epigallocatechin Gallate (EGCG). This is one of the polyphenols (a class of antioxidants) in green tea. Polyphenols in green tea, including EGCG, also help with a host of other things in the body, including heart health, immune health, and cellular repair. Ideally, you want to aim for a green tea supplement that gives you about a six, 6oz cup equivalent per day. So, for those of you who don't have the time to drink six cups of green tea per day, I suggest the brand, NOW, and getting their product called (interestingly enough) 'EGCG'. One capsule twice per day will give you that approximate six cup equivalent in polyphenol content and a whopping approximate eight cup equivalent in EGCG content. Further, this supplement has very little caffeine content. The average 6oz cup of green tea has between 20-30mg of caffeine. If you decide to drink your green tea (ideal), go for the 'Sencha' type, which uses young Japanese green tea leaves. There is less caffeine, and it has more benefits, as the Japanese generally steam dry the leaves whereas the Chinese usually pan dry the leaves. Now, don't anyone get mad at me! These are only general statements. The only negative side to green tea capsules is you must take them with at least some food, as it is acidic to the stomach. However, unlike some other things, once it gets past the stomach, it is actually alkaline to the body as a whole.

Raspberry Ketones: This is another supplement that helps with 'loose fat' burning. The only issue with this supplement is a lot of companies have been found to put very little of the ingredient in their capsules and fill them with red dye instead. This is due to the huge craze that had come out about this supplement a while back, and many companies felt the pressure to cash in. Since it takes around 90 pounds of fresh raspberries to squeeze out 100mg of ketones (the amount in one capsule for many companies), a 'true' raspberry ketone supplement can be fairly expensive to make. A raspberry ketone supplement should cost at least $20 a bottle, otherwise is it likely not legit. There are some other legit ones out there as well, but at this time I would recommend the Eden Pond brand. Take 1 capsule twice per day. That will give you 500mg total per day, which is the dose found to be the most effective. There is no evidence that any more is beneficial. The company also claims their ketones have the highest percentage of adiponectin, the main ingredient responsible for its fat burning properties. Presently, there is a 4 out of 5 stars average rating on amazon with 1722 total reviews.

African Mango: This is a supplement found to be effective at increasing leptin production in the body. Leptins are proteins produced by fat cells which are responsible for getting rid of stored fat in the body. This process is signaled by the brain. The more leptins you produce, the more stored fat turns into loose fat, which is then excreted by the body. Many people, due to their diet, the environment, and hormonal factors, especially women, may be leptin resistant, so they would need something to increase leptin production. The longer a person is leptin resistant, the more fat will store in the body and not get excreted. It will then just keep building and building. Further, when a person is leptin resistant, the brain gets tricked into believing you're hungry when you're not, so you will end up eating more. There are quite a few companies that have come out with an African mango supplement, but from what I've seen, I believe the original is the most effective, which is 'Integra-Lean Irvingia' by Life Extension. Take 1 capsule twice a day.

Coleus Forskohlii: Here is another supplement that has been shown to help with increasing leptin production to get rid of 'stored fat'. This is an Ayurvedic herb that also seems to help with blood sugar and cholesterol balance. For maximum effectiveness, make sure your coleus forskohlii supplement is 'standardized' to 25mg of forskolin per capsule (the active ingredient shown to help with fat loss), and take 1 capsule twice per day (50mg total of forskolin per day) 20-30 minutes before a meal. Watch out, because most coleus forskohlii supplements have very little forskolin, so be sure to read the label. I personally really like the Nature's Plus brand.

Apple Cider Vinegar: Apple cider vinegar helps to liquify both loose food and eventually stored food in your system, so the food get then leave the body more easily. It is also good for helping to kill 'invaders' in your digestive tract, such as bacteria, viruses, and candida; as well as being good for heartburn and acid reflux, as it helps to balance stomach acid. DO NOT take the capsules, as they are just short of worthless. You would need to take about half the bottle for what you would get in just one tablespoon of the liquid. Take 2 tablespoons in 4oz of water 3x/day, 20 minutes before a meal. Do this for 3 weeks, followed by a 5-day break. Then you can do up to 2 more cycles of the same. After that, wait about 2 months and repeat those 3 cycles of 3 weeks on, 5 days off. You can also take apple cider vinegar (same amount and ratio of 2 TBSP in 4oz of water) when you've just eaten too much. You should feel better in about 20 minutes. Finally, if you feel you've just eaten something where you may get food poisoning, you can do it up to 5 times a day, or every 3 hours, but not for more than 2 days in a row. The same goes for when you feel an illness coming on. DO NOT take if you have issues with your esophagus.

Coconut Oil: Coconut oil is a 'good fat' that can help with speeding up metabolism through stimulating the thyroid, as well as burning the 'bad fat' and eliminating it from the body, which can also help with cholesterol and triglycerides. Further, the lauric acid in coconut oil can help with killing viruses, and the caprylic acid in coconut oil can help with killing candida. You must get the raw, 'virgin' type for it to be at maximum effectiveness. (Even though some companies put 'extra virgin' on the label for marketing purposes, unlike olive oil, 'virgin' and 'extra virgin' are exactly the same when it comes to coconut oil.). Also, get one that comes in a glass bottle, as there is a bit of a fear that the acids in coconut oil can possibly cause some of the plastic to leak into the oil. Same as with apple cider vinegar, the capsules are virtually worthless, as it would take way too many to equal what's in a tablespoon. Please note, whether it's a solid or liquid when you see it in the jar, it is fine. 76 degrees is the point where above it turns into a liquid state, and below it turns into a solid state. This is also why coconut oil is a 'good' saturated fat, because in order for it to harden inside your arteries, your body temperature would have to be below 76 degrees, and as we all know, we'd be dead way before our temperature got that low! For weight loss, start with 1 teaspoon twice a day, and increase slowly (every 4 days or so), until you reach 2 tsp 3x/day. For viruses and candida, increase slowly up to 1 TBSP 3x/day for 30 days.

CLA: Standing for Conjugated Linoleic Acid, this omega 6 fatty acid from safflower oil, can help with getting rid of loose fat when it's warm. In other words, in order for this supplement to work at maximum capacity, you must increase your body temperature, either by exercising or by some other means, such as going into a Far Infrared Sauna (FIR), incidentally, the only type of sauna I recommend. Take 1000mg 3x/day right after exercising or getting out of the sauna. Or you can take 1500mg 2x/day, but do not exceed 1500mg at one time. Also, don't take it within 4 hours of going to bed, otherwise it won't work nearly as well.

PGX: This is a patented fiber formula, made by Natural Factors, that has been shown to promote weight loss by detoxing the body of excess food, suppressing appetite by giving you that 'full' feeling (due to the fiber), and even helping with blood sugar balance. Originally, it was only in the form of capsules, and now it's also in packets, as well as in a meal replacement powder formula. Take this whenever you know you won't be able to eat for a while, as some people say it's keeps them full for up to 6 hours! You can also take this as an everyday supplement, but don't make it a habit to eat less times per day than what is ideal for your body. Follow the instructions on the label.

Green Coffee Bean: Green coffee bean extract is another supplement that helps burn loose fat, as well as carbs, while helping to balance blood sugar. It is the Chlorogenic Acid in green coffee bean extract, not the caffeine, that helps with weight loss. Therefore, make sure you get one that's been decaffeinated, at least by around 95%. Get one that's 800mg of the extract per capsule, standardized to 50% Chlorogenic Acid (400mg) per capsule, and take 1 capsule twice per day 20-30 minutes before a meal. The potential side effect with this product is that it can cause a burning feeling or pain in the stomach for some people, as it is acidic. Discontinue if that happens with you.

A couple of notes: First, out of the African mango, green tea, green coffee bean, coleus forskohlii, and raspberry ketones supplements, take only two out of those at any given time, one 'stored fat' burner, and one 'loose fat' burner; such as: African mango and green tea; or coleus forskohlii and raspberry ketones. Then you can switch off to the next two after a couple of months if those aren't giving you the results you desire. You don't want to overwhelm your body, especially your liver. Allow up to one month to notice a difference in weight loss, but it may be sooner. Also, if you take the garcinia, only take one other of the above supplements with that. The food supplements you can take along with the supplements I just mentioned, such as apple cider vinegar, coconut oil, CLA, and PGX. Secondly, there are carb blockers, such as Phase 2, aka, white kidney bean extract, as well as fat blockers, such as chitosan. While these work, I do not recommend taking them, as the also block the nutrients from absorbing, which can over time create nutrient deficiencies. A good alternative to white kidney bean extract is gymnema sylvestre, an Ayurvedic herb that helps break down carbs, almost liquifying them, so they get used for energy instead of getting that blood sugar spike. This also helps with blood sugar balance. Take two capsules 15-20 minutes before a meal that contains carbs. And the best alternative to chitosan would be the apple cider vinegar, as it will break down and liquify the fat.

Endocrine Supportive Supplements

The information in the rest of this chapter will not only help you keep the weight you lose off PERMANENTLY, but it will also help you restore your entire health, body and brain, back to its maximum capacity. So, please pay close attention, as this will tell you EXACTLY why you're not as healthy as you can be, and how to fix it FOR GOOD!

So, here it goes: First, as we discussed before, the best way to tell if there's something wrong with any part of your endocrine system, whether it's your thyroid gland, adrenal glands, pituitary gland, and/or your hypothalamus gland, is whether or not you have low body temperature, as these are the glands that directly (hypothalamus) and indirectly (the other glands) regulate body temperature. When you wake up in the morning, before eating or drinking anything, if your body temperature is below 98.2, you have low body temperature. This is VERY common nowadays, with all the stress we have and chemicals, including heavy metals in our food, water, and environment, as well as the way our food is processed. We've already discussed all the ways low body temperature can affect us and our health at the end of Chapter 2. So, how do we restore our endocrine system so that our body temperature goes back up between 98.2 and 98.6 first thing in the morning?

The first step is to find a Naturopathic doctor in your area and get tested for all the conditions discussed in Chapter 2. This is because these are the most common factors that wreak havoc on our endocrine glands, especially our thyroid. But remember, all of our glands are connected, so when one gets affected, eventually the others will as well if it is not taken care of. When our glands are negatively affected, they can no longer regulate our body temperature properly, as it blocks some of the hormones from being produced at full capacity, and as a result our body temperature goes down and stays there.

Some issues affect our digestive system first and then go to our endocrine system, like gluten (for those of us who can't tolerate it), other foods we can't tolerate, mold, candida, and parasites. Incidentally, mold also affects our respiratory system. Any of these can eventually lead to Leaky Gut Syndrome, especially gluten. And heavy metals, and other chemicals, will affect out endocrine system first, and then go to our digestive tract. The first step to restoring our endocrine system (we'll discuss restoring your digestive system in the next section), is to cleanse our body of whatever issue(s) come up in our test results. You can take a formula for whatever gland is affected all you want, but if you don't clean and restore those glands first, you'll be constantly stepping on the gas and brake pedals at the same time.

If your test shows gluten insensitivity or Celiac Disease, first STOP EATING GLUTEN! There are plenty of books that discuss in detail everything that has gluten in it. Basically, it's in wheat, spelt, rye, and barley. Secondly, take a product called Gluten Ease by Enzymedica and take the maximum dose on the bottle on an empty stomach for at least 2 months, or at least 4 months if it's Celiac. These are specific enzymes designed to eat away the excess gluten that has built up in your body and remove it.

If your test shows a broad spectrum food sensitivity, obviously don't eat those foods any longer until your digestive system is restored (next section), and take a product called Digest Spectrum by the same company, Enzymedica. What Gluten Ease does for gluten, Digest Spectrum does for other food sensitivities. Take it at maximum dose on an empty stomach for 2 to 4 months, depending on how bad those foods have affected your digestive tract.

If your test shows that you have mold in your body, first clean your whole place with a mixture of tea tree oil and water at a ratio of 4 drops of pure, 100% tea tree oil for each ounce of water. You can put it in a spray bottle and spray it around your home, especially the areas that collect moisture, such as your bathroom shower and shower curtain. Next, buy a Nano Particle Silver supplement, such as 'Sovereign Silver', 'Silver Biotics', or 'Silver Sol'. Nano particle silver is way more potent than Colloidal Silver and won't turn your skin blue. Silver is the best thing I know of to kill mold in your body. Take one the silver supplements mentioned above at the therapeutic level amount listed on the bottle for 2 months if no symptoms, or 3-4 months if you have symptoms, such as headaches, extreme fatigue, vomiting, abdominal pain, or respiratory problems.

If your test is positive for candida, get the product 'Candidase' by Enzymedica (no, I do not receive any money for recommending their products; they just happen to make really effective products for these issues). Take 2 capsules, 3x/day on an empty stomach for one month. You will also need a good probiotic to restore the good bacteria in your gut. The best, in my opinion, is 'Healthy Trinity' by Natren. If you can't afford that one, you can get the Garden of Life 'Raw Probiotic' with 85 billion for 3 capsules. This should be taken indefinitely, at a cycle of 4 months on, 1 month off. Of course the first 4 months are the most important. For Healthy Trinity, take 2 capsules a day for the first 6 days, then 1 capsule a day. For Raw Probiotic, follow the directions of 1 capsule 3x/day.

If your test shows parasites, there are many natural parasite formulas out there that work well, but in my opinion, the most effective is Dr. Hulda Clark's regimen. You can find it at the following link: http://www.cleansehelp.com/checklists/hulda-clark-herbal-parasite-cleanse/ A probiotic should also be taken with this, as well as all other healing protocols mentioned in this book for maximum effectiveness of whatever protocol it is. And for those of you who say, 'what about digestive enzymes?' You're right! Those will also help any protocol be more effective. I don't believe there's any reason to spend $25-$40 on a fancy enzyme, when 'Essential Enzymes' by Source Naturals is just as effective in my opinion.

If you test positive for heavy metals, your Naturopathic doctor will go over the best protocol to clean them out, based upon which heavy metal(s) you've tested positive for. Specific supplements are ideal for cleaning out specific metals in your body. But generally speaking, Zeolite in my opinion is the most effective broad spectrum metal binder, which will get most metals out of your system. But again, in this case it would usually be wiser to address the specific metal in your system and what is the best at getting it out. Your Naturopath will know which one you should use and how long to take it. Generally speaking, it takes about 3 months to completely cleanse your body of heavy metals, as they need to be pulled out of your tissues and cells, not just the blood, and that takes some time. But again, the time frame depends on the specific metal. Some examples of heavy metals are cadmium, lead, mercury, and arsenic. If you get Zeolite, I would recommend the one by 'Health Force'

Finally, if you test positive for Leaky Gut Syndrome, that means you've probably also tested positive for at least Celiac and many other food sensitivities. These foods, especially gluten, eventually break down the intestinal lining and get into the blood after they've reached a toxic state from not being able to be eliminated by the body through the digestive tract, which is how it's normally supposed to happen. Toxic state means the food has been sitting in your system for long enough to start collecting 'invaders', usually bacteria, but depending on the food it can also collect fungus and/or mold. Leaky gut is one of those 'syndromes' that unfortunately the mainstream medical community doesn't recognize as legit. This often times will get diagnosed as Chronic Fatigue Syndrome, Fibromyalgia, Colitis,

27

chronic IBS, or Chron's (digestive autoimmune disease).

The first step to healing Leaky Gut Syndrome is to restore the intestinal lining. It will do very little good at this point to take regular digestive repair supplements, as they will only be absorbed at a very low percentage, due to the breakdown of the intestinal lining. This is also why people with Leaky Gut become malnourished. The nutrients are being absorbed at a low percentage. How do we heal the intestinal lining. First, just in case I need to say this again, STOP ALL FOODS YOU ARE SENSITIVE TO. Next, thankfully there is a supplement   that can help restore the intestinal lining. It's called (go figure) 'IntestiNew', and it's by Renew Life. Take 1 scoop twice a day (as it says on the bottle) for at least 6 months, depending on how much damage there is. Yes, I'm sorry, I wish I had a way to heal the intestinal lining sooner. Due to the damage, it takes time. Do not get the capsules, only the powder, as you'd have to take a ton (not literally) of them to equal what's in a scoop. Also add one of the probiotics suggested above (preferably 'Healthy Trinity', as well as a good digestive enzyme, such as 'Essential Enzymes'. If you have pain in your joints, also add a good systemic enzyme, such as 'Wobenzym' by Garden of Life, or 'Repair Gold' by Enzymedica, as these will help eat away the toxic buildup in your tissues, which is what's causing the joint pain. Take at the therapeutic dose on the bottle. After 2-3 months, when you start to notice a positive change in your symptoms, add aloe vera juice with the product 'Aloe Gold' by Aloe Life, at 2oz 3x/day on an empty stomach, or add 'Serovera' instead, an excellent freeze dried aloe supplement, available online at www.serovera.com and follow the directions on the bottle. Either of those you will most likely have to do for 4-6 months. Finally, also after you start to notice positive changes in your symptoms, add MSM powder, by the brand 'Super Good Stuff'(which you can get online at: www.supergoodstuff.com)--(you have to be careful, as many brands of MSM contain toxins), and take 2000mg 3x/day, for 3-4 months, as this will help rebuild the Celia (little hair-like fibers that 'sweep' the food along the digestive tract). I know this is a lot of info, so once again, if you have any further questions, don't hesitate to contact me via the info at the end of the book.

Once you've taken care of whichever issues you had above, it is now time to address your glands directly. Hopefully, you doctor listened to you when you told him/her that you want both a full thyroid panel and a full adrenal panel, or sent you to an Endocrinologist to have those tests done. If not, don't worry, for 2 reasons. First, you can also order any of these, or any other tests, at www.lef.org This is the website for the company, Life Extension. They also make nutritional supplements. Just look for the tests I mentioned, and order them from the website, or you can always call them to order, or if you have any questions. They work directly with Lab Corp, one of the largest lab companies in the country. Just bring the test order to your local Lab Corp, along with the supplies that are sent to you, and they will do the tests there. They will then send them back to Life Extension on your behalf, so that one of their doctors can read your results to you. The other reason not to worry, is that we can also address all endocrine glands at once, including restoring the connection to the brain, nervous system, and digestive system.

Hypothyroidism (Underactive Thyroid) with no Hashimoto's: There are several supplements out there that help to restore thyroid function. If it's your thyroid that is causing your low body temperature, then this may be all you need to restore your temperature to its normal range. One of my favorites is 'Thyrosense' by Dr. Dennis Wilson. You can read more about his founding of the term, 'Wilson's Temperature Syndrome' on his website at: www.wilsonssyndrome.com Then you can get the product at: www.wtsmedproducts.com Generally speaking, you would take 2 capsules twice a day for the first 2 months then drop down to 1 capsule twice a day for the next 2 months. You should start to notice your body temperature going up by at least a half a point after the first month (if your temperature was 97.1, it should go up to at least 97.6), then the rest of the way to 98.2-98.6 after the second month. If you notice no difference at all after the first month, then your issue is most likely not your thyroid. This is why the tests mentioned above are so important, so you're not guessing. The only exception to this is if your T4 is EXTREMELY low, in which case you'll also want to add a raw thyroid glandular supplement. I like the one by American Biologics. They are a highly trusted raw glandular company. Take 1 tablet per day in the morning, preferably on an empty stomach.

Hypothyroidism With Hashimoto's: Since Hashimoto's is an autoimmune disease, we do not treat it in the same way as regular Hypothyroidism. This is because your thyroid will respond differently, and the iodine in the thyroid booting products can actually make Hashimoto's worse. To address Hashimoto's, we need to take care of the digestive portion of the disease, as well as the immune portion. Due to this fact, there needs to be a combination of an excellent mushroom based product for the immune system directly, along with an excellent aloe-based digestive formula for the digestive portion as it relates to the endocrine system. This will also cover all of the glyconutrients, or polysaccharides, our body needs to restore cellular communication so our body can heal. With that being said, there are a few different options, and you can mix and match one of the following aloe products with one of the following mushroom products. 'Serovera' (aloe), available at: www.serovera.com , 'Immune Assist Critical Care' (mushrooms), available at: www.alohamedicinals.com , 'GlycoBalance' (aloe), available at: www.microhealthsolutions.com , 'MicroShrooms' (mushrooms), available at: www.microhealthsolutions.com 'Digestacure Autoimmune X' (aloe), available at: www.digestqure.com Again, mix one aloe product with one mushroom product. All 4 of these are top of the line, and you can't go wrong with any of them. Then of course follow the directions on the bottle of the maximum therapeutic dose, then you can reduce the amount once you're symptoms are gone, or once your body temperature is restored to normal range. Keep in mind, this combo should take care of your Hashimoto's, but you may also need a couple of other products to restore your body temperature. By the way, this is also the protocol I use for every autoimmune disease, not just Hashimoto's.

Hyperthyroidism (overactive thyroid) with no Graves: An overactive thyroid needs to be addressed differently than an underactive thyroid. Here your T4 is high, as opposed to low, as it is with underactive. We need to slow down the production of T4, so your thyroid can return to normal. I suggest a few different methods. As far as food, I suggest eating some type of cruciferous vegetable every day. It would be most wise to go with the ones your metabolic test shows are good for you. These include: Arugula, Bok choy, Broccoli, Brussels sprouts, Cabbage, Cauliflower, Collard greens

Horseradish, Kale, Radishes, Rutabaga, Turnips, Watercress, and Wasabi. These vegetables contain specific types of sulfur compounds, called Glucosinolates. Is there a supplement you can take that contains these compounds? Well, would I be even mentioning it if there wasn't? There are two basic ones, 'Indole 3 Carbinol', and 'DIM'. The best broad spectrum supplement that contains all of these, in my opinion, is 'Triple Action Cruciferous Vegetable Extract with Resveratrol', by Life Extension. Follow the directions on the bottle, and try to eat the foods as well as taking the supplement. There are also other benefits to cruciferous vegetables, such as protecting against DNA cell damage, cancer protection, and the big one, which many of us have but don't know it, too much free flowing 'bad' estrogen in our system. These vegetables help to convert the bad estrogen into 'good' hormones, such as good estrogen, progesterone, and testosterone. Yes, both males and females have all of these hormones. Then the rest of the bad estrogen will get eliminated from the body. Too much free flowing bad estrogen is caused by certain chemicals, especially BPA and other chemicals in plastic bottles that can leak into our water and foods. At the very least, make sure any water or food you buy in plastic containers says, 'BPA Free'.

Other things you can do are eat flaxseeds, and use stevia as a sweetener. Yes, stevia can help slow down the production of T4. Make sure you keep getting tested about once a month to see where your numbers are.

Hyperthyroidism with Graves: Just like Hashimoto's, Graves is a type of autoimmune disease concentrated in the thyroid. Usually, Graves goes with an overactive thyroid, and Hashimoto's goes with an underactive thyroid, but due to the complexity of our 'good ole' endocrine system, this is not always the case. Just make sure you receive a proper diagnosis. As always, feel free to contact me with any questions. The good news is, since the suggestions above for Hashimoto's do not do anything to speed up or slow down thyroid hormone directly, I suggest addressing Graves the same way as

Hashimoto's. In both cases, all we are doing is healing the immune system and digestive system. Doing that will naturally normalize an autoimmune thyroid condition, among other autoimmune conditions, without 'boosting' or 'slowing down' the hormones directly. **Adrenal Insufficiency, high or low Cortisol levels, high or low Adrenaline levels, high or low ACTH levels, high or low Androstenedione levels, Cushing's Syndrome, or Addison's Disease:** Adrenal insufficiency is a broad spectrum term used to describe a situation where your adrenal glands are not functioning properly. Any adrenal condition that does not include an autoimmune component, or a pituitary issue, can be addressed the same way naturally. This is why it is so important to get a full adrenal panel to get properly diagnosed. Most of the time, when we have adrenal insufficiency, it is due to stress, and out cortisol and adrenaline levels will fluctuate. In this case, it is crucial to take an adrenal support product to take the pressure off of our adrenals so they can eventually get back to normal. It's important to note this usually around 6 months or a bit longer. There are quite a few products out there that help, and in my opinion, one of the best is Dr. Dennis Wilson's 'Adaptogen'. Just as his thyroid product, you can get Adaptogen at www.wtsmedproducts.com You can call them at their 800 number if you have any questions. Generally speaking, you would take 2 capsules twice a day for 4 to 6 months, and then 1 capsule twice a day for the next 2 months. You should normally start to feel a difference in about 2 to 3 months. If your adrenaline or cortisol levels are extremely high or low (way out of range), or if they're high or low at all for 2 tests in a row (with getting your tests once a month), you'll want to add an adrenal cortex extract (ACE). One of the best, in my opinion, is 'Sub-Adrene', by American Biologics. Take 5 drops 3x/day under the tongue for 6 months. You can get it at www.americanbiologics.com There is also an 800 number on their site if you have any questions. If you are diagnosed with **Cushing's Syndrome,** which means your cortisol levels are chronically too high, you'll want to make sure it's not due to a pituitary tumor, which is often indicated by ACTH levels that are too high or too low, although ACTH that is too low is more often an indication of **Hypopituitaryism,** or an underactive pituitary gland. If your ACTH levels are normal, I would suggest, after discussing it with your doctor, following the suggestions laid out above for regular adrenal insufficiency. If your ACTH levels are too high or too low, your Endocrinologist must do further testing to see why. Once you have a diagnosis, feel free to contact me, and we'll see what we can do. YOU MUST listen to your doctor and follow his/her instructions in the case of a pituitary tumor, which is rare, which usually means surgically removing as much of it as they can. Finally, in the case of **Addison's Disease,** which is chronically low cortisol production (opposite of Cushing's), you'll also want to know your ACTH levels. Once again, if they're normal, with the blessing of your doctor, you can follow my suggestions above. But if they're high or low, DO NOT do anything until you figure out the reason, and even then this will most likely need medical treatment. Note: Anytime I mention ACTH, the same thing goes for Androstenedione. This adrenal hormone, also included in the full adrenal panel, should also be in range. If it's not, although rare, that can mean a severe issue, often times an adrenal tumor. Don't do anything until talking to your doctor and following his/her advice on what to do about it. Since endocrine issues can be severe, I must say LISTEN TO YOUR DOCTOR, and once again:

* Disclaimer: Be sure and speak to your medical doctor or other licensed health practitioner and get their blessing before trying any of my suggestions. The statements and suggestions I mention in this book, including but not limited to the foods and supplements, have not been evaluated by the Food and Drug Administration and are not intended to diagnose, treat, cure, or prevent any disease.

Underactive Pituitary Gland, Underactive Hypothalamus Gland: If your thyroid gland and/or your adrenal glands are not the culprit of your low body temperature, then it's either your pituitary gland or your hypothalamus gland, and healing whichever one(s) it is will restore your body temperature to within the normal range. You will know that by having those thyroid and adrenal tests suggested above, as well as following the protocols that were laid out. The most common cause of low body temperature is the thyroid, but again it can be one of the other endocrine glands, or a combination of more than one of them. No matter what, get those tests done I suggested by a Naturopathic doctor, and address any of those issues first that come back positive.

As I mentioned, Hypopituitaryism (underactive pituitary gland) can be tested via the ACTH test. If it comes back low, you most likely have it, but once again there can be more serious reasons behind a low ACTH result, so you must find out what's really going on with your doctor. If your Endocrinologist won't do it (a regular doctor will almost never do it), you can buy the test from Life Extension, at www.lef.org Again, this test is part of the full adrenal panel. If your ACTH is off, your Cortisol will almost always be off as well. Having tests on your pituitary and hypothalamus that come back out of range are very rare, but naturally addressing these glands through process of elimination is very safe if you do it in the way I suggest.

Pituitary Gland: The first thing you can do is get a raw pituitary gland supplement. It must be one that's pure from a trusted company. I trust the American Biologics brand. Take 2 tablets once per day in the morning with breakfast. Take it for a month, and if you don't notice any difference in your body temperature in that amount of time, stop taking it, as it's most likely not your pituitary gland that's the issue.

Hypothalamus Gland: Same thing here. With this one, porcine (from pig) seems to be more effective than bovine (cow). I suggest the brand 'Nutricology'. It's expensive but well worth it if it works. The cheapest I've found it is at www.vitacost.com Take a capsule per day in the morning with breakfast. Stop after a month if you notice zero change in your body temperature.

Finally, as promised, I will now reveal a supplement to you that can help restore all communication between the brain, endocrine, and digestive systems in just one supplement. It is called 'Genesis Gold'. In most cases, this will be the ONLY supplement you'll need to take, with the exception of if any of your Naturopathic doctor suggested tests come back positive, if your cortisol or adrenaline levels are WAY out of range, or of course if some kind of endocrine tumor is found. You'll want to take care of those first, then move on to Genesis Gold. Otherwise, you will most likely be able to get away with taking ONLY Genesis Gold. I wanted to give all of you all the information available, as well as a choice of how to address the issues you've found or suspect you have. You may choose to address the issues you have separately, or as a whole with Genesis Gold. It's entirely up to you. Once again, as always, if you have any further questions, don't hesitate to contact me. You can get Genesis Gold at: www.genesisgold.com (I know, go figure) If this is the only thing you do to restore all communication through the three major systems (by the way, I include your immune system in your digestive system), then you will probably need to take Genesis Gold for a year in order to restore your entire system back to 'normal' (the way it was before anything began to affect you.) Yes, it's expensive but of course WELL WORTH IT.

Acid/Alkaline (PH) Balancing Supplements
There are many ways to restore PH in the body, but I really only need to give two options. Ideally, the best option is to get a very high quality green foods powder. I personally recommend 'Perfect Food Raw' by Garden of Life, as it's one of the very few raw greens food powders, which makes it even more alkaline to the body. But if that one is too expensive, there are plenty of others you can get that are of high quality at a good vitamin store. Most of them, depending on the brand, you'll want to take 2 to 3 scoops per day in divided doses. Perfect Food Raw I would recommend 2 scoops a day (one scoop twice a day). It would benefit you greatly to get the unflavored kind (it's really not that bad tasting), as that will be the most potent. I probably don't need to tell you how many additional benefits taking

a green foods powder will have on your body besides just alkalizing it.

If, for whatever reason, you don't want to take a green foods powder, then you can get 'Aerobic 07' by Aerobic Life. This is a stabilized oxygen product that will alkalize you fairly quickly, usually within a month, depending on how acidic you started out at. Take 8 drops 3x/day in about 6oz of water. Do this until both your saliva and urine PH is within normal range, then back off for awhile and pick it up again when you start to become acidic. Remember, you can also be too alkaline, which will cause problems of their own. There is one other excellent way to alkalize your body. This is the most preferred way, as it will not only alkalize you, but it will also give you all the oxygen you need for every cell in your body to thrive. It is alkaline water. It is near worthless to buy alkaline water in a bottle. By the time the water gets to you, it has lost almost all of its alkalinity and has turned into 'regular', or neutral water. The best thing to do is get an alkaline water machine. One that I really like, which is still expensive but way less than the others and works just as well, if not better, is the brand Tyent. It has 2 alkaline water settings, 1 neutral water setting (for when you're eating food or taking supplements or medications), and two acid water settings, for cleaning, beauty water, and watering plants. This machine also filters the water to remove all impurities. This water is great for rebuilding the immune system as a whole, fighting the aging process at a cellular level, and of course helping you lose weight by detoxifying the body as well as bringing your PH levels back to where they should be. Just a reminder to take your PH levels at least once a month to make sure you're not getting too alkaline. At that point, drink the neutral water until you start to drop back into the acidic level. Start with the low alkaline setting until your body gets used to the water (as it can create a detox effect), and then move to the high alkaline setting. Aim for 1/2 your body weight in ounces per day. Again, only drink the alkaline water on an empty stomach, as it will neutralize your stomach acid, and food and other things won't break down properly.

Drink the neutral water with food, supplements, and medication. You do not need the stabilized oxygen drops in addition to the alkaline water. But it is always a good idea to take the green foods power no matter what else you're doing. You can get a discount on it by purchasing the Tyent machine from Diane Underwood at Reverse Aging Naturally. Her number is on her website, which is: www.reverseagingnaturally.com Incidentally, if you can afford it, she also has a top of the line green foods and total nutrition powder, from the brand Purium. It replaces almost every single nutrient. But again, it's quite expensive, so stick with my suggestions above if it's too much for you.

Digestive Support Supplements
We've already gone over many of these in the Endocrine section, as once again, your endocrine and digestive systems go hand in hand, but here is the way to restore your digestive system on its own, in which you may or may not need to add the other supplements from above, depending on what's going on with you specifically.
Step number one: here, we need to talk about the fact that NOTHING else you do will work to its full capacity until your bile ducts are unclogged. Bile is produced by the gallbladder and liver and is responsible for breaking down your food once it gets to the gallbladder and then to the liver. If your gallbladder has been removed, then it puts much more pressure on the liver, as it now has to do all the work on its own. When the bile ducts are clogged, food (and supplements) will not get broken down properly, so they won't be nearly as effective in the body. This can also cause problems in your other digestive organs, as they now have to focus on breaking down your food, which takes them away from their primary jobs. As a result, this will wear them out faster, and you can imagine all the things that can happen if this goes on for too long. So now, you guessed it! The first step to restoring your digestive system is to unclog your bile ducts. And this also goes for EVERYTHING else.

Do the following supplement BEFORE you do ANYTHING else that I've suggested in this book.

Dr. Salar's Liver & Gallbladder Cleansing Salt: You can order this at the following link: http://www.mothernaturesremedy.net/shopbymanufacture/dr-salars/dr-salar-liver-and-gallbladder-cleansing-salt.html Please call Mother Nature's Remedy first to make sure they have it in stock (the number is on the website). If not, ask for the number to order it direct. (I was the one who got it into their store). The directions for use are also on the page where the product is. It is not essential to do the prior week's preparation before taking the product, although helpful, (which is only a 16 hour protocol). You can pick up from where it says, 'Do not eat or drink anything (except water) after 2pm on the day of the cleanse.' Also, when it gets to the part with the olive oil, you can do the 4oz if you want, but I believe 2oz is sufficient, unless you know you have gallstones; then you'll need the 4oz. Plus, that much olive oil at one time can make you vomit, which defeats the purpose. It WILL make you go to the bathroom; that's the point, so be by a toilet! Do not do this cleanse if you're allergic to sulfur. Contact me in that case, and we'll figure out another option.

Step 2 to restoring your digestive system is a full intestinal cleanse. Two days after the liver/gallbladder salts, get a product called 'Mag07'. You can get it online or at many vitamin stores, primarily Vitamin Shoppe and Natural Grocers. Take 5 capsules at night on an empty stomach for 10 straight nights. YES, it will make you go to the bathroom, so be by a toilet! This will cleanse your entire digestive tract including scraping matter off the intestinal walls. That's where this differs from other products. The other way it differs is it does not use harsh herbs, so you shouldn't get those side affects you can get with other products. All this contains is ozonated magnesium. Don't take this if you have kidney disease. Again, contact me and we'll find another option.

Finally, step 3 is to take 'Serovera' for 4 months if you have no major digestive issues, or 6 months if you do, along with the other stuff I've suggested from other chapters. Besides Serovera, at the very least, you should also take one of the probiotics I recommend, along with a digestive enzyme supplement. Again, you can get Serovera at www.serovera.com This is what will help to restore your digestive system. The probiotic and enzyme can be bought online or at several vitamin stores.

A couple other quick notes: Steps one and two (gallbladder salts and Mag07) should be done once every 6 months. Also a liver cleanse and kidney cleanse should be done once every 6 months as well. First, for your kidney cleanse (by the way, only do one cleanse at a time), I recommend 'Kidney Factors' by Michael's Naturopathics. Take 2 tablets 3 times a day for 20 days, followed by a 5 day break, then do another round of 2 tablets 3 times a day for another 20 days. This will help refresh your kidneys. Then, for your liver cleanse, I recommend 'Bupleurum Liver Cleanse' by Planetary Herbals. Start with one tablet twice a day, and slowly go up by one tablet every four days, until you get to 2 tablets 3 times per day (6 total). Once you get there, stay at that dose for 8 weeks. This will help to cleanse and restore your liver.

Brain Restoring Supplements

Remember when we were discussing having too much cortisol, which reaks havoc on the body, creating stress and physical ailments? Well, did you know cortisol is also concentrated in the brain? Too much cortisol in the brain also causes stress, anxiety, depression, loss of short term memory, and eventually brain disease. The largest symptom of too much cortisol in the brain is foggy thinking. How many of us can relate to that? But not to worry, my little grasshoppers. There is a supplement that can help calm brain stress by helping to remove excess cortisol out of the brain. It's called Phosphatidylserine (PS). This is a nutrient our brain already makes, but the more stressed we are, the more gets stripped out of our brain. This nutrient is fairly expensive, and may need quite a bit of it, but you will feel a world of difference after just a couple weeks of taking it. The standard dose to feel a significant difference can be anywhere from 300mg to 800mg per day. You also must take it in dividing doses, especially at first, otherwise it can make you tired until you get used to it. It also needs to be in softgel form, as it is fat soluble, with the patented 'Sharp PS' symbol on it. It should also be taken with food that contains at least 5 grams of fat.

The good news is there is one brand that meets the criteria that is not overly expensive. It's the Swanson brand, 100mg, with 90 softgels in the bottle. They make more than one type, so make sure you get that one. Start with 1 softgel 3x/day (300mg total). Wait two weeks, and if don't notice enough of a difference (you'll notice some), then increase to 2 softgels twice a day (400mg total). That amount should make a pretty significant difference, but if you feel you still need more, you can increase it to 2 softgels 3x/day (600mg total). It is very rare that someone would need more than that, and you should never exceed 800mg/day total.

If you need additional brain support, there are a few excellent brain formulas that work very well and address all areas of proper brain function. One of my favorites is 'Clari-T' by Life Seasons. It's fairly expensive but well worth it, especially when you consider you'd pay at least twice as much if you bought each ingredient separately. You may have to search online a bit to find the best price, but from what I see now, amazon seems to be the cheapest place to get it. Take 1 capsule twice a day. Clari-T does have 50mg of PS in it, so adjust your dose of PS by itself accordingly.

Everyday Recommended Supplements

There are a few supplements I recommend people take on a regular basis. First, you need to request a blood Vitamin D test from your doctor. Many doctors still don't get the fact that Vitamin D is vital for just about every function in the body. You are asking for disease if your Vitamin D levels are considerably low. Ideally, your blood

Vitamin D level should be between 50ng/ml and 80ng/ml (nanograms per milliliter). The amount of Vitamin D you should take daily is a direct relation to how low you are, as well as how much sun you plan to get to help raise your levels. A good maintenance dose, if you get very little sun is around 2000IU per day. The amount should be raised just for the time you're low, and can be anywhere from 3000IU to 10000IU per day. It is very rare, unless someone is under 20ng/ml that I recommend more than 5000IU per day, and even then, no more than 5000IU should ever be taken at one time (if you do 10000IU, it should be in divided doses and only for a short time, such as one month.) This is because there is a danger to raising your blood calcium levels too high, which will wreak havoc on your parathyroid gland (the little gland that sits right behind the thyroid gland). This can cause irregular heartbeat, and will eventually begin to affect the thyroid gland, and then the other glands. How ever much you take, you should repeat the Vitamin D test once a month. As soon as your levels are within the range listed above, drop down to 2000IU per day. Vitamin D must be in either a softgel or liquid, as it is fat soluble, and should be taken with food that contains at least 5 grams of fat. Ideally, you should get as much of your Vitamin D from the sun as possible. Start with 10 minutes per day of direct sunlight, and increase gradually to 30 minutes of direct sunlight per day. The worry of skin problems comes when we get more than 30 minutes per day of direct sunlight, between 10am and 2pm (the time when the sun is the strongest). Any more than that, is when you'd want to start using sunscreen. Also, unless you have diagnosed eye problems, do not wear sunglasses (but don't look directly into the sun either), as much of your immune system is controlled by how much sun gets into your brain through your eyes. This is also is how much of your serotonin is produced and regulated. If you have any questions about how much Vitamin D you should be taking, contact me.

The next nutrient you want to get on a daily basis is magnesium, another nutrient (in this case a mineral), that every cell needs in order to properly function. Aim for somewhere between 600mg and 750mg per day total, including a combination of food and supplements. Most people don't get very much magnesium from food, so keep that in mind. No more than 250mg of magnesium should be taken at one time, as your body will not absorb it all.   Don't go over 750mg per day, as it can affect your kidneys. Magnesium supplements should either be food based, liquid, or in the form of Aspartate, Asportate, Glycinate, or Malate. The Citrate form should only be taken if you're using it at night to help you sleep, for leg cramps, restless legs, or to help you go to the bathroom. The Oxide form should not be taken, as it is poorly absorbed, and the carbonate form should not be taken, as it will bunch up in the body, almost like a rock.

Next on the list is calcium. In a perfect world, a Calcium/Magnesium combination supplement would contain the proper ratio, as well as in the proper forms of each mineral. Unfortunately, from what I've seen, that world does not exist. Let's make this simple. The best calcium supplement, in my opinion, is 'Bone Strength Take Care' by New Chapter, as the calcium comes from algae. It also contains other naturally occurring minerals that can help to heal the bones from the inside out. 'Raw Calcium' by Garden of Life is also top of the line, and very similar to Bone Strength Take Care. You can't go wrong with either one. Just be sure to adjust your Vitamin D and magnesium supplements accordingly, as those supplements also have those nutrients in them. If those are too pricy for you, the only other calcium form you should be taking, besides food based, is the Citrate form. Never take the Carbonate form, as this will bunch up in your system and eventually cause calcium stones. If you eat or drink quite a bit of dairy, I suggest around 500mg per day as a supplement, in two or three divided doses. If you eat little or no dairy, then around 250mg 3x/day (750mg total) is what I suggest. Somewhere between 800mg and 1200mg total per day, including all sources, food and supplements, is what to aim for. Any more than 1200mg, and especially more than 1500mg can cause heart palpitations and be dangerous over a period of time.

Next, we have a Multiple Vitamin/Mineral supplement. This should definitely be food grown. Unfortunately, the vast majority of MultiVitamins, as well as all other vitamins, are synthetic or at least have a synthetic component. There are a few brands I recommend that are food grown. They are 'New Chapter', 'MegaFood', 'Garden of Life Raw Vitamin Code', 'Garden of Life My Kind' (even better because it's organic), and 'Country Life Real Food Organics'. Most of them have different ones for different ages and genders. I highly suggest getting one where you take more than one per day, as the one-a-day's are not enough to get all of the nutrients you need. Also, if you get one that has less than 250mg of Vitamin C, I suggest you add a food grown Vitamin C supplement that puts you somewhere between 250mg and 500mg per day. Multi-vitamins should be taken at a cycle of 4 months on, 1 month off, as your body gets used to them and then they're not as effective.

Ok, next we have fish oil. Most of us do not get enough omega 3 fatty acids in our diets alone. If you already eat a 'fatty' fish at least 3 times a week, then it is not necessary to add a fish oil supplement. Examples of this are salmon, mackerel, sardines, herring, dark tuna (without the fat removed), anchovies, trout. Please be sure to contact the company you're purchasing the fish from and make sure they contain non-detectable levels of mercury. Egg yolks, flax seeds, chia seeds, and hemp seeds also contain omega 3's that are good for us, but they don't have enough of the DHA we need for the brain, or enough EPA, which helps with proper heart function. Incidentally, the other great component of eggs yolks is the choline, which not only delivers essential nutrients to our brain, but it also helps break down the cholesterol in the yolks, as well as the bad cholesterol in our liver, which is one reason the cholesterol won't affect us negatively, unless we go way overboard. One more point about that is you would have to eat quite a bit of cholesterol for it to raise our cholesterol levels in the body. It's the animal fats and trans-fats (from hydrogenated and partially hydrogenated oils) that raise our cholesterol. Ok, back on track with fish oil. As a supplement, you want to aim for around 600mg per day of DHA, and around 850mg per day of EPA. One of my favorite fish oil supplements I recommend is 'Elite Omega 3' by Carlson. Not only to they purify their fish oil as well as any other company, but unlike most other companies, they do not use heat to do it, so all of the nutrients remain in tact. All you need is 1 capsule twice a day to get the amount of DHA and EPA you need. Back to eggs for a moment. The ideal amount of eggs to eat in a week is between 4 and 7, organic, cage free, of course. If you don't eat eggs, a great way to get the choline your brain needs to function properly is from Lecithin. The granules are the most convenient. Take 1-2 Tablespoons per day, ideally 2 TBSP, 1 twice a day. You'll want to mix it with food, as you need to chew it first for it to break down properly. Make sure the Lecithin you get is non-gmo.

Now there's probiotics and digestive enzymes. A good probiotic, like one of the ones I've already recommended in this book a few times, should be taken in a cycle of 4 months on, 1 month off. Digestive enzymes should be taken with every meal until your body temperature is back within normal range. At that point, as long as you're eating the raw, organic foods that are recommended for your metabolic type, you should no longer need digestive enzymes, as your body is now producing enough, along with the enzymes coming from the raw foods. However, if you still find yourself eating more than 20% of your diet from cooked foods, you should still take the enzymes with the cooked meals.

Finally, CoEnzyme Q-10 (CoQ-10) is the final supplement I will talk about. CoQ-10 should be taken by everyone over 40. It is responsible for much of our cellular function throughout the body, especially in our heart. Take 100mg a day of the hydro-soluble (Q Gel) Ubiquinone form from age 40-50, then go up to 100mg twice a day from age 50-60, and finally after age 60, switch to the Ubiquinol form and take 100mg twice a day. After age 60, our body loses much of its ability to convert Ubiquinone into Ubiquinol. On the flip side, if you start taking the Ubiquinol form when you are too young, your body will just waste a lot of it. A good hydro-soluble CoQ-10 is made by Country Life, and it's called 'MaxiSorb Mega CoQ-10'. When you get to the point of needing the Ubiquinol form, there are many brands available, and as long as it's from a trusted company, you'll be ok. Make sure to buy it from a vitamin store, not a drug store. As an example, the brand Jarrow is a good choice.

* Disclaimer: Be sure and speak to your medical doctor or other licensed health practitioner and get their blessing before trying any of my suggestions. The statements and suggestions I mention in this book, including but not limited to the foods and supplements, have not been evaluated by the Food and Drug Administration and are not intended to diagnose, treat, cure, or prevent any disease.

CHAPTER 5
Different Exercises for Different People

The first thing I'll say is although I do know quite a bit about exercise as a whole, this is an area I would not consider myself an 'expert' at. I will however be able to give you the basics; enough to where you should have at least most of the information you'll need. Now that that's out of a way, I'll start by saying that everybody is different. Different people need different types of exercise for their particular body type, and you need to find the exercise that works best for you. Having said that, I will definitely give you some guidance.

The only complaint I have about the metabolic typing results I've highly recommended in this book that you get by taking the test, is that it doesn't include which exercises are best for different metabolic types. But there is some good news. The book 'Eat Right 4

Your Type', by Dr. D'Adamo, does go over the best exercises for different blood types. Make no mistake, EVERYONE should be doing some type of exercise everyday. Without movement, our muscles become weak, and we die sooner. It's as simple as that. Not to mention, we will have a heck of a hard time losing weight.

What does exercise do for us? (1) It helps speed up metabolism, as well as helps control appetite via our hormones, so we lose weight faster. (2) It improves circulation, which helps with blood pressure, blood sugar, cholesterol, our immune system, stagnation, coagulation, and overall health. (3) It strengthens the heart and all other muscles. (4) It greatly improves the detoxification process through sweat, circulation, removing stagnation and coagulation. (5) It helps boost our mood by increasing various neurotransmitters. (6) After a while, it gives us more energy overall, helps us sleep more deeply, and makes it so we don't need quite as much sleep.

Before I get into various exercises, I'd like to mention one way to vastly improve the results you'll get from exercise. Not only will this therapy help with that, it is also the single most important thing you can do to detoxify the body and improve your overall health, including dramatically slowing down the aging process. It's called a Far Infrared Sauna. It is the ONLY type of sauna you should ever use. It uses dry, infrared heat, which it exactly what our body functions on, including all of our cells and organs. If you have a place by where you live that has a far infrared sauna, get yourself a membership there and use it. If not, even though it's expensive, it's well worth it to buy one for your home. The best deal on the best sauna you can get is with Diane Underwood at 'Reverse Aging Naturally'. Go to her website at: www.reverseagingnaturally.com and give her a call. She has one of the very few sauna brands that have no detectable Electromagnetic Frequencies (EMF's), as well as no detectable toxins from the wood that is used. The brand is 'TheraSauna'. If you do find a place by your home that has a far infrared sauna you can use, make sure the brand they have has no detectable EMF's coming from the heaters, and no detectable toxins in the wood used to build the sauna.

* Disclaimer- Consult with your doctor or other licensed health care practitioner before beginning any exercise program or using a Far Infrared Sauna.

Now, back to exercise. There are many people who should be doing non-rigorous exercises, such as fast walking. There are others whose body needs rigorous exercise, such as Tae Bo. Use the blood type book as a guide, and do what works best for you. Ideally, the general rule of thumb to achieve the maximum benefits from your exercise routine, if you only do cardio, is 45 minutes of rigorous exercise, or 1hr and 30mins of non-rigorous exercise. Any more than that can overwork both the heart and the immune system. Exercise should be done right upon awakening if possible, as this will set your metabolic rate for the day. If you do aerobic (cardio) and anaerobic (weightlifting), the anaerobic should be done first, as the first 20 minutes of exercise only burns carbs, so by the time you get to the aerobic exercise, you're now burning fat. Further, if you do both, weightlifting should be around 30 minutes, followed by another 30 minutes for rigorous cardio, or about another hour for non-rigorous cardio. It would be very wise to hire a personal trainer, so he/she can conform a routine that's specific to your goals and for your specific body type.

CHAPTER 6
The Mental Part of Weight Loss

Besides being a Certified Holistic Health Practitioner, as a Certified Hypnotherapist I can tell you without a doubt that the mental part of weight loss, especially keeping it off, is just as important as the physical part. I've worked with hundreds of clients in hypnotherapy just for weight loss alone, and I can not tell you the transformations

I've witnessed. It literally transforms your mind into believing there is never a reason to eat unless you're hungry, as well as stopping the second you know you're about to be full, and knowing exactly when to eat a sweet food to treat yourself, as opposed to a craving. It also commits your mind into exercise and living healthy as a whole.

I do holistic health & healing consultations over the phone, all over the country. As far as hypnotherapy, it is very important for at least the first session (preferably all sessions) to be face to face. I can always do your holistic consultation over the phone, and if you'd like to do hypnotherapy, I can recommend a good Hypnotherapist for you in your area if you contact me. Of course if you live near me, I can do your hypnotherapy sessions as well.

If it's not convenient or feasible, money wise, to go to a Hypnotherapist, I will now give you a good alternative method on how to make sure you stay on track with losing the weight and keeping it off for good. It is a self-hypnosis method, and just like anything else, it will take quite a bit of

practice, especially in the beginning. I highly suggest that you record the session below into a tape recorder and listen to and follow along with it that way. Also, I suggest you do this once a week for the first 3 weeks, then once every 2 weeks for the next 3 times, then once a month for the next three times. After that, I would do it once every 3 months 3 more times, then you're done. Ideally, you'll want to actually see a Hypnotherapist, so he/she can progress the following sessions as needed for where you are at that time. But like I said, the self-hypnosis session below is a good alternative.

Start by sitting in a comfortable spot, preferably a spot you don't sit very often, even at someone else's place. Do not do this on your bed. Pick a spot on the wall in front of you, or if you're outside, pick a spot in the air or a building in front of you. Allow yourself to stare at that spot and notice the spot getting more and more blurry, your eyes getting more and more tired with possibly a redness, dryness, or burning sensation. The urge to blink becomes greater and greater, but at for least for now fight that urge. Notice yourself wanting to be calm and comfortable and wanting to relax more and more. Now begin counting backwards from ten down to zero. With each count, notice yourself wanting to go into deep relaxation more and more. Count slowly... ten... nine... eight... seven... six... five... four... three... two... one... and tell yourself SLEEP!!! Now feel yourself drifting down more and more... more and more... more and more... Now you'll begin counting backwards from five down to zero. With each count, feel and allow yourself to drift down even more, knowing at zero you'll will have reached the deepest part of self hypnosis you can achieve today. This is where all the positive changes you've ever wanted will now happen. Five... four... three... two... one... and tell yourself SLEEP! Feel yourself drifting down even further for another ten seconds in complete silence, and if it hasn't gotten there already, your mind is now completely clear, and your body is completely limp and loose, like a rag doll. You will now make a written contract in your mind's eye with your subconscious mind, that each and every suggestion you give yourself will be taken into the deepest part of your subconscious mind, immediately and literally, and will be immediately used for your greater good beginning NOW and lasting your entire lifetime. Now, tell yourself there's a reason you've held onto your reasons for not losing the weight you've wanted to, and not having the health you've wanted to, up until now. But it is that same reason you are here NOW to break that barrier and get to your ideal weight, and to your ideal health. You now know with every fiber of your being that NOW is the time. Now, picture or imagine yourself standing at the top of a hill or mountain at your ideal weight. There is a mirror there that you brought with you. Look into that mirror and notice you can't help but have the biggest smile on your face that you've ever had in your life. THIS IS YOU in the near future. You've now seen it; you now KNOW it. Now, go back into your mind and notice some things have changed. You're now completely committed to dropping the weight you've always wanted. Having the health you've always wanted. Now, visualize or imagine a large hollow ball next to you.

Notice now that all of the reasons you haven't dropped the weight up until now are drifting into that hollow ball, more and more... more and more.. more and more. All the thoughts, feelings, emotions, actions, reactions, beliefs, old patterns you now no longer have. Now, count backwards from seven to zero, as that allows the remainder of those old reasons to finish drifting into that ball. At zero, that ball is going to lock with all of those reasons in it. Seven... six... five... four... three... two... one... and LOCK IT!!! As you can see, there is no way those reasons can escape the ball, no matter how hard they try. Now, notice that ball with all of those reasons begin to drift away, farther and farther... farther and farther... farther and farther. When you say 'GONE', you will you longer be able to see that ball, and it is at that exact moment you know that ball is gone forever and will never come back. See it drifting farther... farther... farther... farther... and now say GONE!!! And notice the relief; the weight lifted off your shoulders, knowing it's completely gone. Now, come back into your mind and notice your mind beginning to fill up with up with positives. Your mind has to replace what used to be there, so once again, notice it now filling up with only positives. Positive thoughts, positive feelings, positive emotions, positive beliefs, positive responses, positive actions. Now, counting backwards from six to zero, noticing with each count all those positives getting closer to locking into the brain forever. At zero, you'll find yourself saying the word 'LOCK'. So now counting backwards at six... five... four... three... two... one... and LOCK!!! Now notice how all those positives will not escape; EVER. They are there to stay. Now, notice yourself going through your everyday life. No cravings; eating ONLY when you're hungry; stopping the SECOND you begin to feel satisfied. Exercising, with your exercise of choice, every day. Drinking all the fresh, clean water you know your body needs. Knowing you can treat yourself every once and awhile, having complete POWER over it. Now, you'll be counting upwards from 1 to 5. With each count you'll find yourself getting closer to the waking state, until at 5 you are completely awake, refreshed, alert, and ready to take on the world as your best self. Now beginning to awaken at one... noticing once again where you are at two... and excellent sense of health and well-being at three...beginning to really awaken now at four. And now at FIVE! Eyes open, WIDE AWAKE!!

Final Thoughts

My plan is to always over-deliver on all my promises. I sincerely hope I've done just that with this book. I hope it was worth way more to you than what you paid for it. I have the exact same mentality with my clients, spending as much time with them as it takes to help them heal. Although I'm absolutely entitled to make a good living with what I do, as I truly am one of the best there is in the industry, I also don't believe in gouging people. I deliberately charge considerably less than other so-called 'famous' natural health practitioners.

My goal in this book was to cover as much as possible when it comes to losing weight and healing yourself of whatever ails you, partially, but greatly, by understanding the reasons most of us get sick and hold onto weight in the first place. Although I am fairly certain I can help you heal from whatever it is that ails you, physically and/or mentally, when you contact me with any questions you may have, although I may 'encourage' you a bit, because I know I can help you, as I have thousands of clients previously, I can absolutely promise I will not 'pressure' you into making an appointment for a session. I'm certain that I was not able to cover 'everything' in this book, as that would be impossible, but again I truly covered as much as I could, and for anything else, please don't hesitate to contact me with any questions you may have. Finally, we all need to realize that things are constantly changing in the natural healing industry, including even better products coming out in the future for helping to heal from various health conditions, so feel free to contact me to inquire about the 'latest and greatest' that has come out at the time you've read through this book.

With that being said, here is my website and contact info:

Jason Teichner, CHHP, CN, CHT

www.healhealheal.org

lookfeelbehealthy@yahoo.com

(775) 527-7791

* To Your Health and Happiness; Let's walk this path together! JT

Further Reading:

Stop The Thyroid Madness by Bowthorpe, Why do I Still Have Thyroid Symptoms by Kharrazian, The Thyroid Cureby Corey, Tired of Being Tired by Hanley & DeVille, Adrenal Fatigue by Wilson & Wright, and From Fatigued to Fantastic by Teitelbaum, Eat Right 4 Your Type by Dr. D'Adamo. Food Combining Made Easy by Shelton, Therapeutic Exercise: Foundations and Techniques by Kisner & Colby

References:

Chapter 1

http://www.theguardian.com/lifeandstyle/2013/feb/20/a-history-of-diets-byron-52

Chapter 2

http://www.innerbody.com/image/nervov.html

https://www.blendspace.com/lessons/sDtiZcOo3BnBhQ/the-digestive-system

http://www.scientificamerican.com/article/gut-second-brain/

Chapter 3

http://thegarciniacambogiaextract.org/hca/what-is-hca-in-garcinia-cambogia/

Chapter 4

http://idealbite.com/raspberry-ketones/
http://dictionary.reference.com/browse/Leptins
http://www.allnaturalprevention.com/pages/heavy-metal-toxins.htm
http://www.cancer.gov/cancertopics/factsheet/diet/cruciferous-vegetables
http://www.nlm.nih.gov/medlineplus/adrenalglanddisorders.html
http://labtestsonline.org/understanding/analytes/acth/tab/test
http://labtestsonline.org/understanding/analytes/acth/tab/test